Help!
My Diet Sucks!

CHRIS JANKE-BUENO

ISBN: 9781701790285

DEDICATION

To my wife and kids. It's been my dream to have a family of my own since I was a young kid. I'm blessed to have this life. You guys rock!

CONTENTS

CHAPTER 1
ANOTHER DIET BOOK?!?

Most diet and nutrition books present a new "cutting edge" way to eat in order to be the new miracle cure for weight loss and all things healthy.

They usually present information that we somehow missed in all the years that we've been studying nutrition. How did we ever expect to get healthy without this new information?

But the path to health is not cutting edge. We've known about how to get healthy for years, even decades. We know there are no "get fit quick" schemes that actually work. What works are healthy choices over a period of time.

What works is a checklist.

Most people do not need the newest research on the subject of nutrition, they need to practice the basics, and continue to refine their behavior until those basic habits become ingrained in their life.

New Habits. New Health.

This book is about modifying behavior, not about the latest and greatest "secret" to health.

There are no secrets. And if there are no secrets, then you have all the tools right now to achieve your health goals. Yes, right now! There are no more excuses. No more waiting. Now is the time to act. Let's take one step at a time, together.

About The Format Of This Book

This book is meant to be practical. So the general format of the book follows more along the lines of a checklist that you would put on your refrigerator.

The book is simply a detailed version of the checklist. For the printable PDF copy of the checklist that you can hang on your refrigerator, visit www.ChrisJankeBueno.com/checklist.

Feel free to read the whole book, but you don't really need to (not all at once at least). The only thing you need to focus on is the one part of the checklist that you are on. You might find that you haven't even mastered step one, and that's fine. Stick to step one until you really feel like you have it mastered.

The book is designed so that the steps build off of each other. Step one is the most important step because it creates a domino effect to all the other steps. Likewise, step two is the next phase in that progression. So as tempting as it might be to go out of order, try to follow the steps as they are presented. There is a reason, and it works.

Motivation For The Journey

It's very likely that you will lose motivation along the way. it can happen even to the most motivated among us. Nobody can maintain 100% motivation at all times for a goal that takes months or years to complete. Even professional athletes must be highly aware of their emotions, and make corrections when they sense the slightest dip in motivation.

So what do you do to keep your motivation high? There are lots of strategies that can work. One that I like is beginner's mind. This is where you approach a practice as a first-timer. Beginner's mind is an extremely effective way of approaching life in general, and this goal in particular. Always look at your daily habits with fresh eyes. How would you look at this habit of yours on the first day?

Human beings follow habitual tendencies in order for us to be effective in our day-to-day lives. For example, if you had to consciously think about how to tie your shoes every time you did it, you would use so much brainpower on that task that you would not be able to think of much else. Habits go to our subconscious, and we don't need to focus on them as much. But if you are overweight and out of shape, you want to shine some light on your habits. Be very mindful of all the actions that you have been doing up until now that have been habitual. We want to take them out of the habit mode as we begin to create new habits.

At first, these new habits might seem weird. They might be challenging. Healthy people do these naturally, and you can too. Once you begin to turn these tasks into habits, you are well on your way to becoming a healthy person.

The key is to focus on the daily habits rather than the final outcome. For example, if you change your habits in 60 days, but you still have 100 pounds to lose in total, just know that you have achieved success with the habit formation. The weight loss is just a matter of time. Continue doing what healthy people do and you will have what healthy people have.

I know from experience. I have been overweight myself. And I know that in order to become healthy, you need to first begin thinking like a healthy person, and then begin acting like a healthy person.

Sometimes it's challenging to think like a healthy person if you don't feel healthy. In that case you might need to adopt the "fake it till you make it" mentality, meaning that you might just need to start with the actions on this list and soon you will start to feel healthy. In that case the feeling will follow the action. If you do the actions enough then eventually you will feel healthy.

CHAPTER 2

THE 4 STEPS TO PERMANENT CHANGE

Through the process of going from unhealthy to healthy, you will walk through four separate stages. Each of these is necessary in order to get to our final outcome of automatic health. Pay close attention, and see if you can identify which phase you're in now.

Step 1 - Unconscious Incompetence

In this phase, you don't even know that you're not good at something. It's not even on your radar. You don't know what you don't know. Consequently, you make no effort to improve, because you're not even aware that there's anything that might need improving.

You've likely used the phrase "ignorance is bliss." That's phase 1 for sure. If you're in phase 1, you are probably very content. So why leave? Why try to get to step 2 and beyond? That's a good question, and ultimately one that only you can answer.

For me, I like to ask the questions, "what don't I know" and "what am I missing here?" Both questions will get you out of any stuck patterns of looking at life, and open you up to more productive mindsets.

The key to getting out of this step is awareness. Just waking up to new ways of looking at the world will take you out of this step. This first step can be painful, because all of a sudden you're going to realize what you don't know.

Step 2 - Conscious Incompetence

Once you learn how you can live a better life, you may feel simultaneously hopeful and defeated. Enthusiastic and depressed. Motivated and guilty.

Why these conflicting emotions? One major reason is that now you know what mistakes you've been making, yet you also may see that correcting those mistakes is the path to a healthy life. But at this point you are so far away from your final destination that you might feel despair.

The good news is that you're conscious. You're aware. You can shine some light on your old habits and ask if they're helping you or hurting you.

I believe this is the most painful part of the four steps, because you are well aware of how poorly you've been doing with your health habits.

But if you can just hang in there for a bit, you will realize that sometimes being a bit uncomfortable is actually a great place to be. This is where learning happens. Change also happens here. Without discomfort, there is no reason to change.

Think of it like this: when you were "unconsciously incompetent" you probably had issues with your body that you weren't even aware of. But just because you were not aware of them does not mean they don't exist. By identifying where you can improve, you can take the first steps to making that improvement.

Step 3 - Conscious Competence

With enough learning and practice you can quickly progress to getting to a place where you can make the right healthy choices… provided you're aware enough to make them.

The limitation here is that you must remain highly conscious in order to implement your new healthy habits. Your tendency is still toward the unhealthy. Yes, you know enough to make the right decisions, if you are thinking about them.

This step is where most well-meaning people get stuck. They think it's enough to simply learn new information. Of course it's a great start, but learning information and living that information are two totally different things.

By the time you have finished this book, you will be firmly rooted in step 3. Be happy about this, and also know that you're not quite done yet.

If you stay in step 3 you will have all the knowledge but not be able to back it up with consistent action. The result will be frustration.

The way to get out of step 3 and into step 4 is through repetition. I have exercised consistently for more than 30 years, yet I still go to the gym. Why? Repetition is the most valuable health skill you can cultivate. Our health is constantly moving, getting better or getting worse. And if you're not putting in the effort to get better then you are getting worse. Make the decision to constantly improve by repeating your habits over and over again.

Step 4 - Unconscious Competence

You've practiced these habits so much that they've become a part of you. You don't even have to think about them anymore, and so you can go unconscious.

Does this mean you can relax your standards and start eating fast food? That's actually a trick question, because someone who is unconsciously competent has healthy habits that are so rooted that fast food doesn't even cross their mind. Here's an example of what I mean. I notice that many people who give driving directions use landmarks to tell others where to go. Sometimes those landmarks include fast food restaurants. I've lived in San Jose, California for 37 years and realized that there were fast food restaurants that I drive by weekly but I didn't even know they were there because they are so outside of my reality. I've achieved unconscious competence in that way.

I'd like to show you one last concept to demonstrate an important point to you. You've likely heard the expression that it takes 10,000 hours of practice to get good at something. This is also true of healthy habits. To give you an idea, if you divided those 10,000 hours into an average 40-hour work week, it would take you 250 weeks to achieve that expert level of mastery. That's five years!

I say that because I want you to be realistic. If you're a fast-food-eating, soda-drinking type of person, don't expect these long-term habits to go away overnight.

But you can change, and you can get healthy. It takes time. It takes effort. But you can change your life and your body.

Are You Ready?

I hope that you are actually a little bit nervous right now. Some nervousness would show that you know that some big changes are about to take place. But think back to your first day of school when you were a kid. Most likely you were nervous for a day or two, but then once you got to know some people and realized that this new year would not be very scary, you started to settle in.

The same thing will happen with this. At first it will feel strange, but these healthy habits will begin to feel like your own. You need to stick with it long enough for this to happen. Whatever it takes, never give up on yourself. Never ever give up! You can do this!

I'd love to hear your progress along the way. If you're open to sharing, Drop me an email at Chris@MyCoreBalance.com. Feel free to also join me on YouTube and Facebook.

I have been a personal trainer since 2004, and one of the things I love about it is seeing results from people. As an author, I don't get to see you. It would mean the world to me if you reached out with your questions, comments, and story. Not just for me, but for others like you who could benefit from your story.

Thank you for trusting me to guide you on this journey. I feel so honored and privileged to be coaching you through this seven step process. Right now it might feel overwhelming, but I know that soon you will refer to it as the simple seven step process.

Here we go.

Trust the checklist!

CUT ALL BEVERAGES EXCEPT WATER. DRINK ½ TO 1 GALLON PER DAY.

If you're not drinking enough water, it doesn't matter how healthy your diet is, you are not getting one of nature's most vital nutrients. That's why we want to start with water.

Another reason is that often times when we think we are hungry, we are actually thirsty. If we follow what we think is hunger, then we end up eating food that our body really didn't even need. This is just extra calories that will make weight loss more challenging.

Many people are overweight and out of shape because they drink so many calories. The unfortunate thing about this is that most drinks are not going to fill you up. So you have a double negative here: you have high calories and no satiety. Meaning you will tend to drink more than you want to.

When was the last time you felt satiated drinking a soda? Yet, a soda contains so many calories. The more you eat over your expenditure, the more weight you will gain. This includes *drinking* calories as well.

So there are two parts to this first step. First, eliminate all liquid except water. Second, drink at least half a gallon of water per day, working your way up to a full gallon per day.

You might say, one gallon is so much water! How am I ever going to manage this? Don't worry, you'll be fine. This is absolutely doable, you just need to change your habits. Slowly, steadily, and at your own pace. This is not going to happen overnight.

You are right if you're thinking that you will be peeing a lot. You will, at least at first. A doctor friend of mine described what happens when somebody begins to increase their water intake.

The kidneys of a dehydrated person are similar to a dried out sponge. If you have a sponge on the countertop, you can still use it even if it's dried out, but you will need to run some water over it.

If you have ever done this, you know that that sponge does not absorb the water right away. It takes a little bit of time and you waste a lot of water in the process, but gradually it starts to absorb and retain that water. The same kind of thing is happening with your body. You do not have the capability yet to absorb all the increased amount of water that you're drinking. So, your body does what it is supposed to and pees it out.

Keep drinking more anyway. Eventually it will level out.

Make sure that you have this habit firmly rooted in your day. Make sure that you give this habit your 100% full focus for at least a week, longer if needed. Once you feel like the habit is a part of you, then you can begin to think about moving on to the next step.

HABIT 2

DRINK YOUR GREENS DAILY

I know, I know. I told you that the only thing you can drink is water. Here is the only exception. And it is a requirement that you consume some sort of green drink every day.

Once you have significantly raised the bar with the quantity of water that you drink, you are ready to fine-tune that water intake. The next step is to add water-rich vegetables into your day. This comes in the form of a green vegetable drink.

Nobody in the history of diet books has ever said that vegetables are bad. The only problem that people typically have is consuming enough of them in their raw form to really make a difference in their overall health.

The green drink is the best way that I know to get enough vegetables quickly.

Before you turn up your nose at the thought of drinking vegetables, let me first assure you that the recipe that I'm going to give you has modifications to make it very delicious, even for a non-vegetable fan.

You are already drinking 1 gallon of water per day, you're going to siphon some of that water and pour it into a blender. Then you will add some fruits and vegetables, and blend yourself a daily drink.

Here is the recipe. Stick with this, even if you have tried other ones. This is the most basic and foundational low-sugar green drink that has helped hundreds of my clients lose weight.

Alexis had been training with me for four years. She lost 30 pounds in those four years, but she still had 10 more to lose. After months and months and months of me harping on the importance of adding a green drink to her daily diet, she finally agreed to try it. **Within one month she lost the 10 pounds.**

This recipe is powerful!

My brother-in-law always played sports growing up but never had a six-pack. Despite being in very good shape, his body fat was never low enough to reveal his abs. **Within two weeks of drinking the green drink every day, you could see his abs.**

This drink is powerful!

I believe this step is one of the most important steps. It helps you to establish a baseline, a standard by which your taste buds function. Once you begin to taste the subtle sweetness of these greens, you are well on your way to eliminating other bad things from your diet. And what's great about that is that it will happen naturally, because you will start to hate the taste of unhealthy food.

The recipe is simple.
- Start with 3 cups of water in a blender (take it from your gallon).
- Peel one lemon and throw it in.
- Add one whole cucumber,
- a small handful of spinach,
- and a whole avocado.

If you are a newbie, you want to make the drink more palatable. You have options. Notice that the first two ingredients, lemon and cucumber, are the same ingredients that most spas put in their water. So with the first two ingredients you are drinking spa water. Everybody likes spa water, right?

The way to make this more palatable is to add more lemon and cucumber, and decrease the amount of spinach and avocado in your drink. I had a client a few years back who literally put one leaf of baby spinach into her green drink because she couldn't stand the idea of drinking vegetables. "That's fine," I said. "Keep doing it every day and soon you will add more, but make sure you do it naturally and not because I told you to." It did take her a while, but within two months she was up to a handful of spinach.

Why the avocado, you might ask? Besides having lots of healthy fat in the avocado makes the mix creamy. Try blending this without the avocado, and your drink will look more like a green beer than vegetable juice. You will have about an inch or two of frothy head on the top of your drink. There's nothing wrong with this, it just makes it harder to drink. And anything that is not super convenient and delicious will not be a habit that sticks around very long. Add the avocado, and experiment with what the right amount is for you.

A note on blenders. I am very partial to the Vitamix. There's no other blender out there who can completely chop this drink up properly. It works. It's by far the best blender out there. Get one as soon as you're able to. Yes, it is an investment, but last I checked they had a seven-year warranty. My Vitamix has lasted me over 12 years. It's worth the upfront cost.

HABIT 3

CUT PACKAGED SNACKS, REPLACE WITH FRUITS AND VEGGIES

Let's talk snacks. I'm not a big fan of snacking, although I do "eat between meals." This might seem like a contradiction, but it's not.

In fact, my goal is to eat no snacks whatsoever. I differentiate between snacks and meals. I would rather have you eat "small meals" than snacks.

What's the difference? In my mind, the only difference between a snack and a small meal is macronutrient breakdowns.

Don't worry too much about macronutrients yet. More details will come in later chapters. Right now, I want you to focus on two main things for your snacks: greens and proteins.

The reason why snacking is so bad the way that most people do it is because it's almost 100% carbs and fat. We are going to flip the script and split our snacks between greens and protein.

Let's keep this simple. Your snack should be roughly one handful of greens and one handful of protein.

- 3 ounces of chicken with five pieces of broccoli? *Great!*

- A half a canna tuna fish with three stocks of celery? *Fantastic!*

- A quarter cup of edamame beans with a handful of baby carrots? *Now we're talking!*

See how easy this is? Snacks are not fancy. No dressings, no flavorings, no fuss. That should be easy. Yes, borderline bland, but so what. Would you rather be fit and eat plain food or out of shape eating your tasty Snickers bar? Let's remember that by now your taste buds have already changed.

So let's add this into our day. Make it easy on yourself. Get a cooler and stock half of the cooler with your protein and the other half with vegetables. Every time you get hungry between meals use your left hand to scoop out a handful of protein, and use your right hand to scoop out a handful of green vegetables. Put it on a plate and eat it.

How many snacks should you eat in a day? Honestly, as many as you want. Just establish the habit. Your body will eventually tell you when you've eaten enough, when it is nourished and satiated. Don't worry about eating too many vegetables, that's impossible.

Give this habit your undivided focus for as long as it takes. Don't let it take too long though. Realistically you can create this habit in the next few days. Get going, it's worth it.

CUT FRIED FOOD, HYDROGENATED OILS, AND TRANS FATS. REPLACE THEM WITH HEALTHY FATS

By the time you get to the fourth habit on your checklist, you are doing pretty well. You have your liquids and food between meals all set. Now, we need to change your meals.

A lot of this might've already happened because again your taste buds have probably changed. That's great! You are ahead of the game.

Unless you've been living in a cave, you know that fried foods are not good for the body. We also want to get rid of trans fats and hydrogenated fats. These are indigestible fats that will just make you fat.

On the other hand, eating healthy fat will actually help you stay lean. That is an essential nutrient that we need to eat in order to survive.

I'm going to make it easy on you. There are five main categories of good fats. Leave everything else alone except for these five categories:

1. Avocado
2. Coconut
3. Olives
4. Seeds
5. Nuts

That's it! Now, do you have free reign to eat as much of these as you want? No, that wouldn't be good. You are going to need to balance these with the rest of your food.

A "handful" of avocado is about ½ to one whole avocado. I handful of olives is about 8 to 10 olives.

Use your best judgment, and if you're finding that you're eating too much, eat less next time. Don't beat yourself up over it, just make the adjustment.

This is the first step: you will actually be clearing out your pantry. Go through your pantry and clear out all foods with The word "hydrogenated" in the ingredients. Any type of hydrogenated oil needs to be thrown in the garbage.

If you feel guilty that you're throwing away food, don't. The stuff is not food. It has a shelf life of decades. Real food doesn't.

Every fat that you eat it must be natural in order for it to be healthy for your body. Get rid of all unnatural fats and replace them with the five healthy fats.

Once you have done that, move onto the next step.

HABIT 5
CUT PROCESSED PROTEIN.
ADD NATURAL PROTEIN.

You're doing great! You are on step five out of seven. Before you go on, congratulate yourself for making it this far. You have developed some solid health habits.

If you feel like any of your habits could use some more development, now's a good time to go back and make sure that those are firmly rooted in your daily routine. Now, let's move onto protein.

Protein is a vital building block to add muscle. If you are participating in a resistance training program, you will definitely need high-quality protein. If you are not participating in a resistance training program, when would *right now* be a great time to start?

Protein is relatively straightforward. If you eat meat, your protein will consist of anything that comes from something that has eyes. Beef, chicken, fish, etc. all come from animals which have eyes. Eggs come from chickens, which also have eyes. You get the idea.

If you are vegetarian, the eyes rule still applies. Milk comes from cows, which have eyes. Eggs from chickens, which have eyes.

Vegans will have a little more trouble with protein. You don't eat anything with eyes. You are going to have to rely on nutrient dense fats and carbohydrates to get your proteins. Most of your protein sources are actually not going to be predominantly protein.

Think of the common vegan proteins. Lentils have protein, but they are mainly a carb source. Nuts have protein, but they are mainly a fat source. So, when adding your protein, you need to be aware that you are balancing your carbs and you're fat. It's not very hard to do, but it will take some practice.

In general, when you're shopping for protein sources, you want to go with organic, free range, grass fed, pasture raised, etc. Words like these are great indicators to indicate the health of the protein.

Also look for phrases like "no hormones added." Of course, manufacturers of these proteins can lie and cheat and "bend" the truth. But if, in general, you are looking for these types of labels, you will more often than not be consuming very healthy food.

Focus for the next few days to weeks on gradually replacing the unhealthy protein sources with healthy protein sources.

You are well along the path to good health.

Once you have mastered this habit, move onto the next one: carbohydrates.

CONVERT FAST CARBS TO SLOW CARBS

Step six. Don't slow down now. Carbohydrates are the last macronutrient that I'm focusing on, mainly because there's so much mystery around them. I wanted to make sure that you have some success with the essential nutrients of fat and protein before we move onto carbohydrates.

Keep in mind that you are getting carbohydrates from your green drink. If you are not working out, this is probably enough carbohydrates to sustain you throughout the day. Again, you do not need concentrated carbohydrates unless you are expending energy above and beyond the typical American workday.

If you are exercising regularly, pregnant, or nursing, this chapter applies to you.

You may have heard the term glycemic index. The glycemic index refers to the spike in blood sugar from certain foods. This is what we will be using to determine whether a carbohydrate is "fast" or "slow."

A fast carbohydrate enters the bloodstream quickly, gives you a huge spike in blood sugar and therefore insulin, and then you crash. Soda, candy, cookies, alcohol, etc. will give you this reaction. Your body hates these things. And once you become acutely aware of the feeling that you get from these carbohydrates, you will too.

Opt instead for slow carbohydrates. These carbohydrates enter the bloodstream much slower, provide a sustained level of energy, and taper off slowly as well. You will not be getting the crash that you do with low carbs.

Lentils, sweet potatoes, oats, vegetables, etc. are all great examples of slow carbs.

Your homework is to search online for "low glycemic foods" and out of the top eight, choose your favorites.

Go shopping and replace all high glycemic carbs with these favorites.

Like the previous steps, you're going to get rid of all food that does not match these criteria. Get rid of your high glycemic carbohydrates.

That's all I have to say about carbohydrates. There have been scores of books written about them, about how bad they are, about how good they are, about how neutral they are. Really, who cares? Just get in the habit of eating slow carbs, and you'll be fine.

Once you establish this as a habit, and you have replaced carbohydrates in your pantry, move on to the last step.

PRACTICE PERFECT PROPORTIONS

It's been quite a journey. You have systematically taken the actions needed to get ridiculously healthy. Don't stop now, you're almost done.

This chapter is about putting it all together. You've done your fats, your proteins, and your carbs. Now, what do your meals look like?

The answer to this question is pretty simple actually. You have your three macronutrients, plus the category of "greens" in relatively equal portions on your plate, each representing 25%.

You already know which foods to put in each of these. This step just refers to the ratios.

This ensures that you are not eating a plate of salmon and nothing else, even though wild caught salmon is very healthy. To the exclusion of everything else, it is not balanced.

You're not going to have a dinner plate full of olives, even though they are a very healthy source of fat. You need to balance it with your protein, carbs, and greens.

This habit is very straightforward. Every meal will have an equal portion of protein, fat, carbs, and greens.

A note about carbs: like we said before, if you are not particularly active, your carbohydrate intake will not need to be as high. In this case, replace your carbohydrate quarter with greens. Instead of rice or pasta, you can eat more kale or asparagus.

Now let's talk about snacks. Remember earlier in the book when I mentioned that a snack should have greens and proteins. Now I'm going to tell you that you should start snacking less and eating more meals. Here's an example: if you eat three meals a day and two snacks per day, try to instead do four meals per day and only one snack.

The only difference between a meal and a snack is the proportions. A snack might be just tuna with celery, but to make it into a meal you're going to add olives and lentils. It doesn't have to be a big meal, but it is balanced now and therefore we call it a meal and not a snack. The entire meal might literally only fit in the palm of your hand. This is the final key to developing winning eating habits.

You might say this seems too easy. You might think that it won't work. I have been around health and fitness for three decades, and I can confidently tell you that there's nothing new under the sun. I've read books written in the 1920's that said the same things that the new "cutting edge" research is touting as the next big thing.

Forget about fads and go with what works. If you're not as healthy as you want to be, use this 7-step checklist as an audit to get back on track.

One habit will lead to the next, and pretty soon you'll have momentum. And I hope you're able to look back and say two things:

1. That was easy, and
2. That was fun!

Enjoy your life! Cultivate your health one step at a time.

ADDITIONAL RESOURCES

Health is an end in itself, yet it's also a means to fully enjoy your life. Now you have a firm foundation on which to stand.

If you ever slip, or "fall off the wagon" as they say, it's no big deal. In fact I can guarantee that you will fall off the wagon. That's great, you're human. You are going to fall back into some old patterns every now and then. This book is short enough where you could read it quickly any time you need a quick checkup.

I hope this book was valuable to you. Thanks for taking the time.

For more resources, visit me at www.ChrisJankeBueno.com

Or information about my fitness business, visit www.MyCoreBalance.com

A MESSAGE FROM CHRIS

First of all, thank you so much for reading this book. I hope it was beneficial for you. As you can probably tell, I'm not really much into the "latest and greatest" fitness or diet craze. I'm a big believer in the basics. The basics work.

Before I became a personal trainer, I majored in history. I love reading about the history of health and fitness. Some of the best books were written 100 years ago, long before supplements and steroids.

Back in the early 20th Century, men and women were building lean, muscular physiques without any enhancements. Just food. Trust me, you do not need the latest and greatest diet or supplement to reach your goals. You need the basics, practiced consistently, for a long enough period of time.

I've been a personal trainer for 15 years now, and I've

seen all the fad diets come and go. But core principles never change.

If you have questions or comments, feel free to message me directly on any of the social media platforms.

And if you are in the bay area, specifically San Jose, come and train with me. I would love to meet you.

Your friend in health,